SUPERHERO

WWW.SUPERHEROSIMPLIFIED.BLOGSPOT.COM

SIMPLIFIED

EST. 2013 CLEVELAND, OHIO

Also by Scott Burr

Fitness and Martial Arts

Superhero Simplified: *Collected, Selected, Revised and Expanded*
Get a Grip*: A Practical Primer on Grip Strength and Endurance Training… and More*

Fiction

Bummed Out City: A Novel
We Will Rid the World of You: A Novel

SUSPEND YOUR DISBELIEF

HOW TO BUILD AND BUILD STRENGTH WITH THE WORLD'S MOST RUGGED SUSPENSION TRAINING DEVICE

SCOTT BURR

SUPERHERO
WWW.SUPERHEROSIMPLIFIED.BLOGSPOT.COM
SIMPLIFIED
EST. 2013 CLEVELAND, OHIO

SUSPEND YOUR DISBELIEF: *How to Build and Build Strength With the World's Most Rugged Suspension Training Device* is published by Superhero Simplified Publications in conjunction with Artless Dodges, Inc.

Suspend Your Disbelief: How to Build and Build Strength With the World's Most Rugged Suspension Training Device
Copyright © 2016 Scott Burr
ISBN-13 978-0-9907227-5-5
ISBN-10 0-9907227-5-9

Published by Superhero Simplified Publications
in partnership with The Artless Dodges Press
Cleveland, Ohio
www.SuperheroSimplified.BlogSpot.com
www.TheArtlessDodgesPress.com

Cover illustration from Bengala No. 23
Drawing credit Los Hermanos Ortiz

Layout and cover design by The Artless Dodges Press. Photos by Jennifer Allanson and the author.

READ THIS FIRST

The instruction and information contained in this manual are no substitute for hands-on, in-person training with an experienced professional. It is advised that before you attempt anything shown or described in this manual you consult with a qualified trainer. Superhero Simplified and Scott Burr accept no responsibility for any injury or death resulting from you attempting anything you read in this manual.

Always consult your physician before beginning any exercise program. The general information contained in this manual is not intended to diagnose any medical condition or to replace the information available from your healthcare provider. It is advised that you consult with your healthcare professional to design an exercise program that is appropriate to your current health and fitness level.

If you experience any pain, discomfort, or difficulty when performing these exercises, stop and consult your healthcare provider.

In this text I employ the universal masculine. This was not done with the intention to slight, marginalize, or offend anyone. I sincerely hope that it will not detract from this manual's usefulness to you.

PART ONE

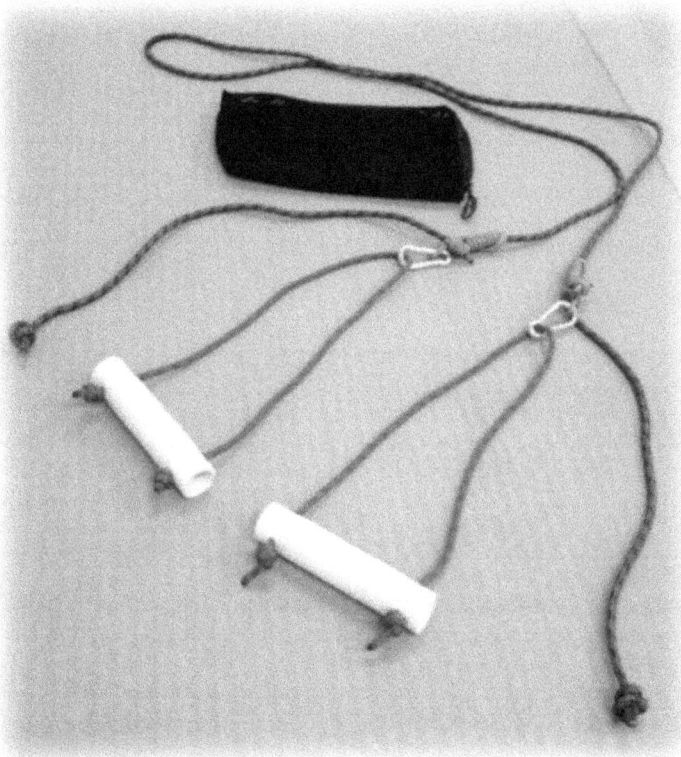

BUILDING YOUR
SUSPENSION DEVICE

CONTENTS

INTRODUCTION

The suspension device described in this manual was designed by Steve Maxwell. It's cheap, easy to build, rugged, lightweight, and extremely versatile. For those of you who know about Steve and his vagabond, road warrior lifestyle, you already understand how everything Steve carries with him has to prove its value or get left behind, and this suspension device is no different (for more on Steve visit www.MaxwellSC.com).

Once the materials are gathered, this suspension device should take no more than 30 minutes to build.

It is my intention that, when used with the instructions provided in PART TWO: YOU AND YOUR SUSPENSION DEVICE: A LOVE / HATE STORY, this suspension device will provide you with everything you need to have a top-level strength workout in under 30 minutes in any type of location or conditions.

ANATOMY OF A SUSPENSION DEVICE

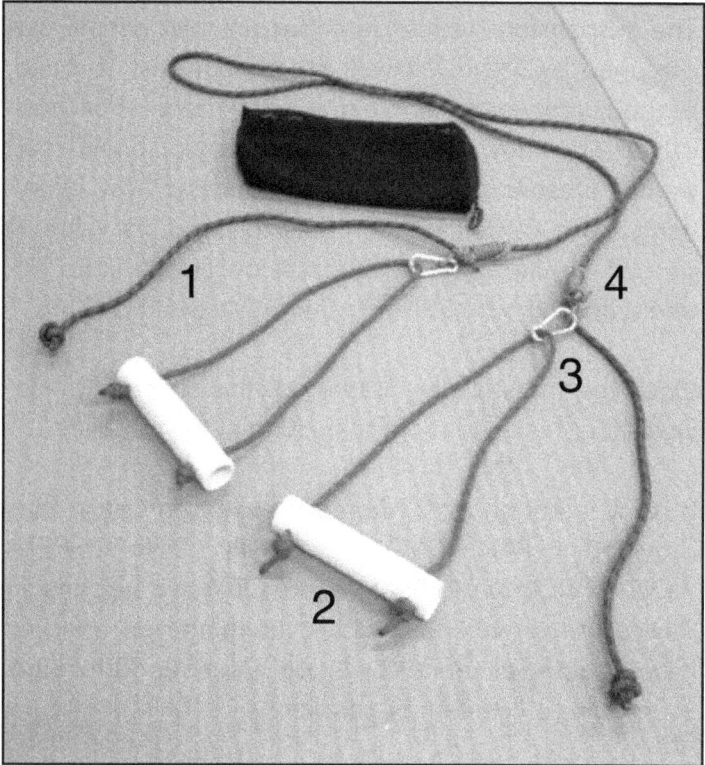

1. Central Cord (7-8mm cord)
2. Handle (1″ PVC, 5-6mm cord, athletic tape)
3. Utility clip (or Carabiner)
4. Prusik Cord (5-6mm cord)tied into a Klemheist Knot

TOOLS AND MATERIALS

The tools you will need to assemble this suspension device include:

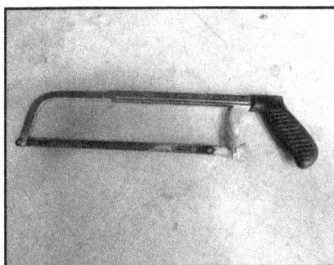

Saw

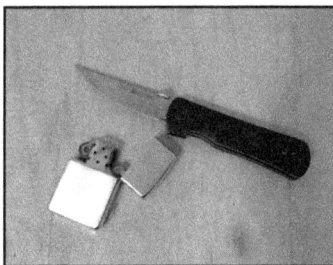

Knife and Lighter

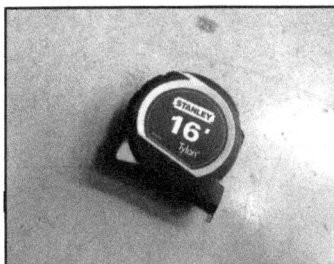

Tape Measure

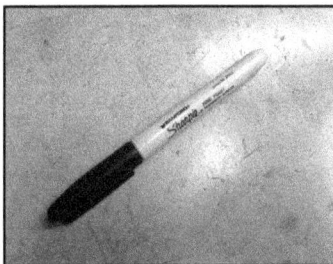

Sharpie

Drill, with a bit slightly larger in diameter than the cord you will be using to make your handles.

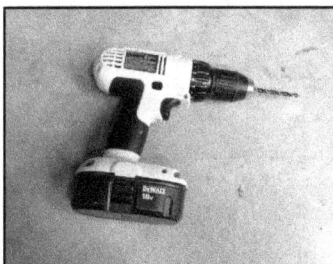

The materials you will need to construct your suspension device include:

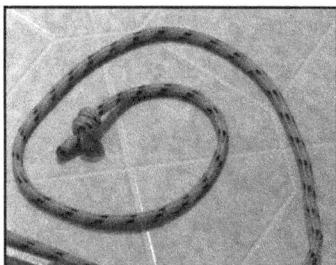
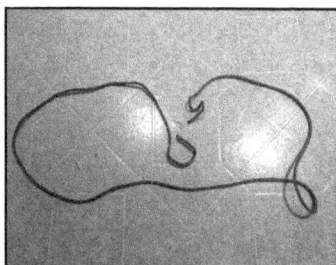

10'-12' of 7-8mm static climbing cord AND 10'-12' of 5-6mm static climbing cord. The 7-8mm cord will form the central cord of the device, while the 5-6mm cord will be used for the handles and prusiks (see: ASSEMBLY). This can typically be purchased at any outdoor gear supply store. The 5-6mm cord will need to be cut into quarters. Two of the strands will form your Prusiks and the other two will be used in the construction of your handles.

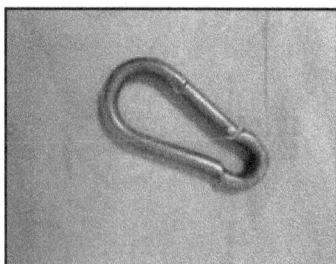
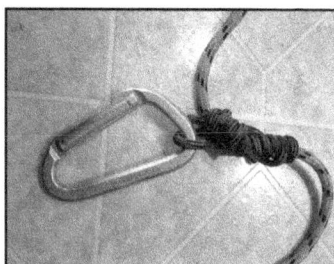

2 carabiners OR hardware store utility clips. For the workout described in YOU AND YOUR SUSPENSION DEVICE, a utility clip with a load tolerance of greater than half your bodyweight but less than your full

bodyweight is acceptable. However, if you plan on advancing at some point to single-limb training, it is advisable to select clips with a higher load tolerance.

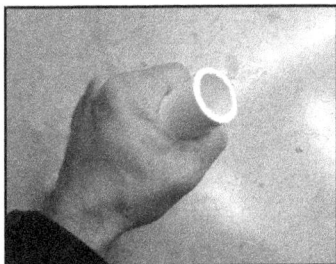

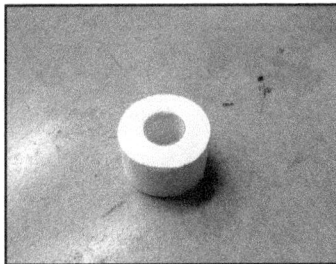

12"-14" of 1" diameter PVC pipe. This will become your handles. If you have large / wide hands you'll want to get a longer piece. The athletic tape is optional, but I prefer to wrap my handles for a better grip.

ESSENTIAL KNOTS

To assemble your suspension device, you'LL need to know how to tie a DOUBLE FISHERMAN'S KNOT and a KLEMHEIST KNOT. The double fisherman's knot will be used to construct our Prusik cord and to finish the ends of our central cord so that our handles don't slide off. The Klemheist Knot will be composed out of the finished Prusik, and will attach our handles to the central cord.

The Double Fisherman's Knot:

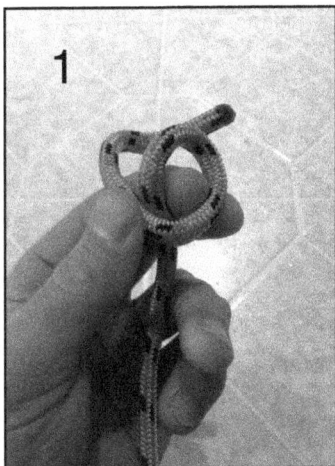

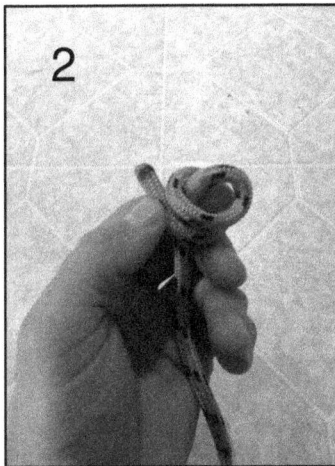

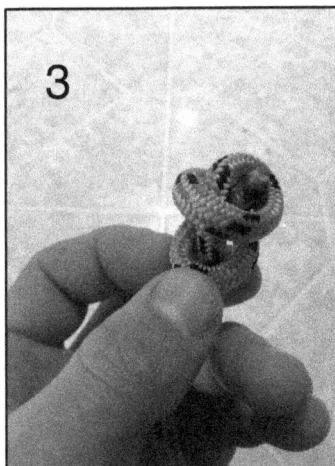

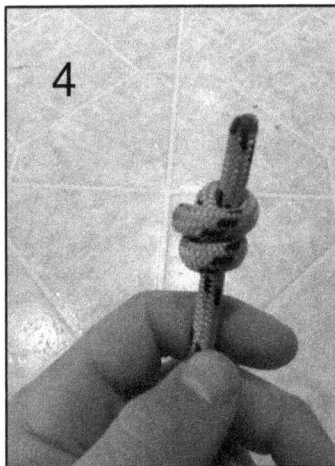

1. Bring the end around the front of the cord to form a loop. 2. Bring the end around the central cord a second time. 3. Pass the end through the loops. 4. Pull tight.

Making a Prusik Cord using the Double Fisherman's Knot:

With one of your 5-6mm pieces: 1. Form a loop with your cord, so that 2. the ends are positioned running past each other. 3, 4, 5. Starting on one side, tie a double fisherman's knot over both strands (the end that is forming the knot and the other line). 6. Do the same thing with the other side, and 7. pull the lines so that the knots slide together. 8. You now have a complete Prusik cord.

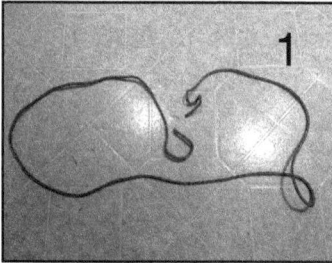

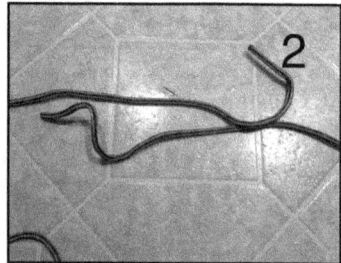

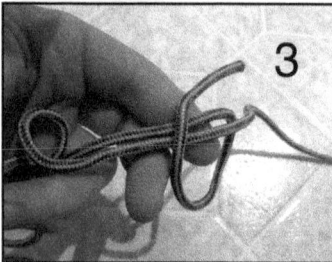

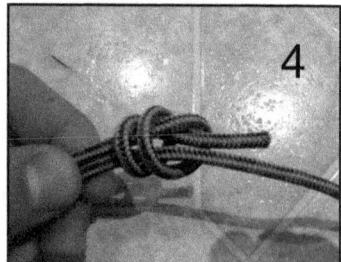

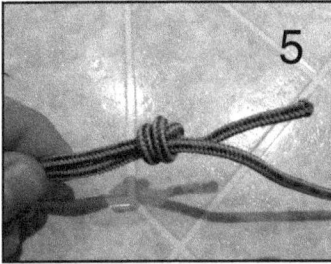

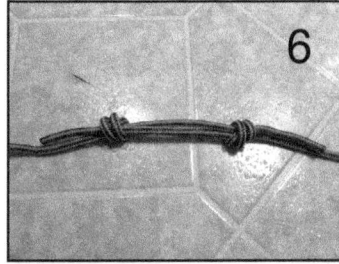

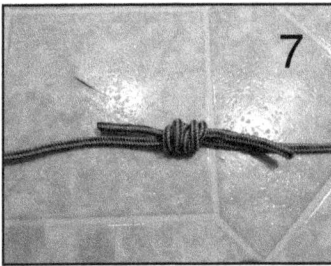

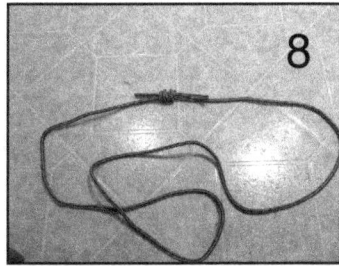

The Klemheist Knot

The Klemheist Knot is a friction knot. It is formed by wrapping a Prusik Cord around another line, in this case the central cord of our device. When weighted, the Klemheist knot tightens down on the central cord and bears weight; when unweighted, it can be slide easily to any position on the line, making it the ideal knot for a making an adjustable device. A description and illustration of the Klemheist knot's action will follow.

1. Lay your Prusik cord under the central line, with the double fisherman's knot at the bottom (toward the end of the central line, rather than towards the middle). 2. Wrap the doubled Prusik over the central line, wrapping toward the middle of the central line. 3, 4. Wrap the Prusik three or more times. 5. Pass the remaining loop through the bottom loop, where your fisherman's knots are. 6. Clip your utility clip or carabiner through the loop.

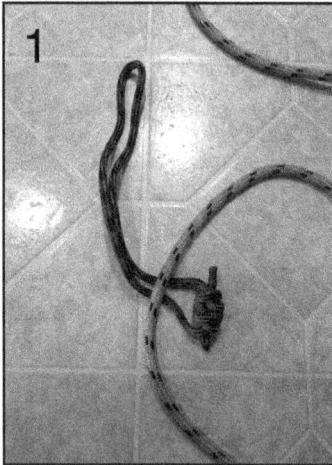

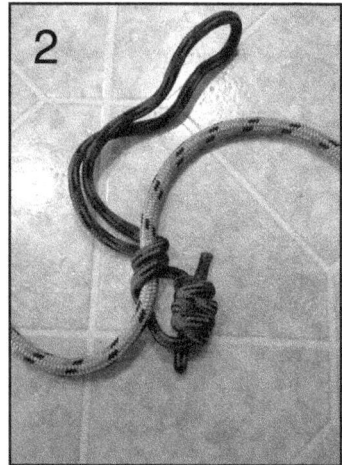

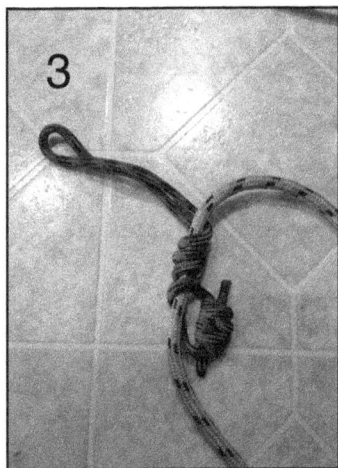

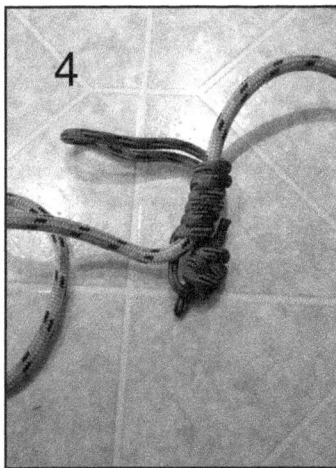

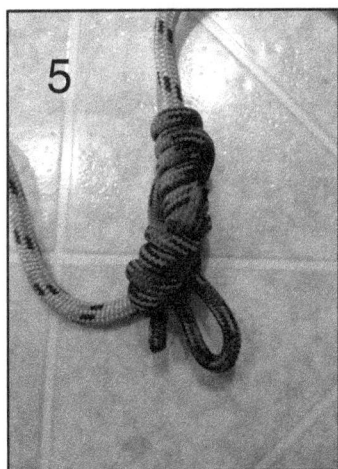

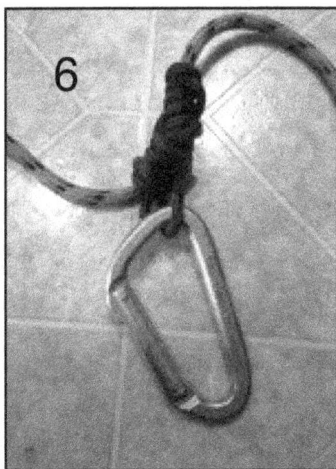

ASSEMBLY

To assemble our device, we need to assemble and finish the component pieces. These include the Handles, the Prusiks, and the central cord.

BUILDING THE HANDLES

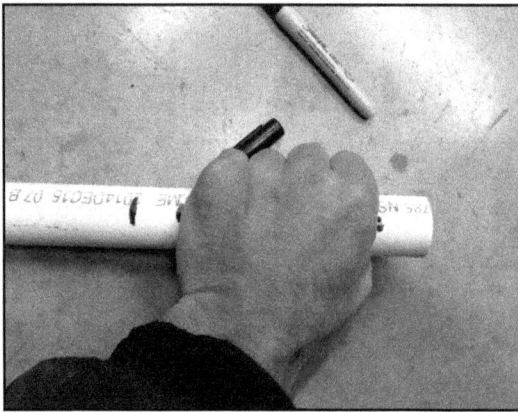

Measure the PVC for your hands. For the average hand each handle need be no more than 6" in length, but make sure this measurement works for you. Hold the individual handle segments in the middle, where you imagine your hand would go, and mark where the edges of your hand are with the sharpie. Note that the handle piece will be longer than your hand to provide room for the cord.

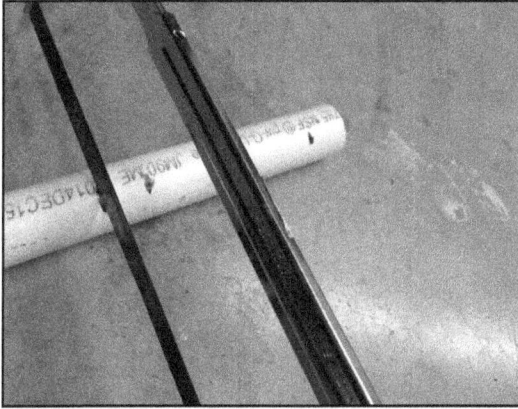

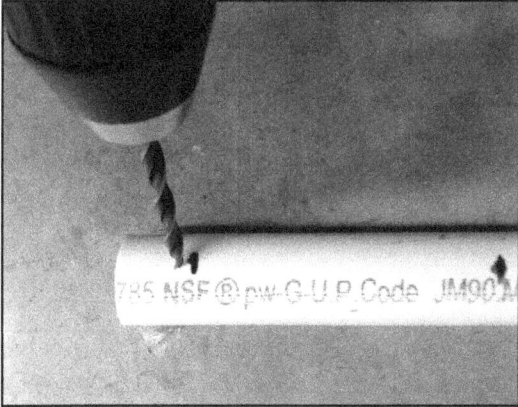

Cut the PVC to length, and drill the holds for your cord. Drill just outside the mark you made indicating where the edges of your hand were. Make sure to leave room on the outside (towards the end) so that the knot has support. Drill through both sides of the PVC in as-close-to-vertical a line as you can.

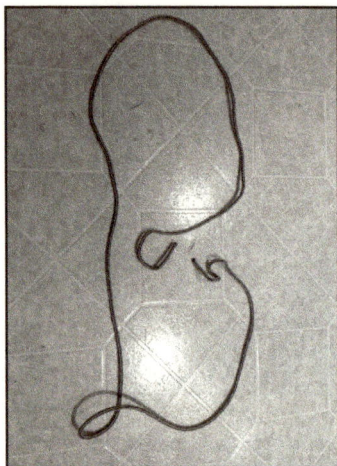

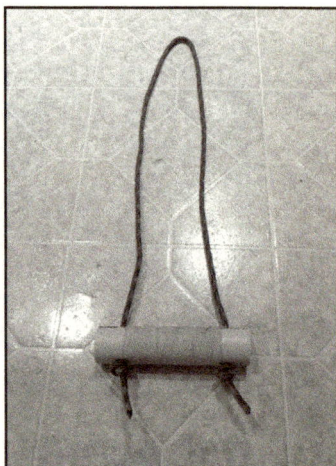

Using one of your 5-6mm cord pieces, pass each cord ends through one set of holes, and tie off with a double fisherman's knot. Wrap the PVC with athletic tape (optional). The finished product should look like the picture on the right. NOTE: make sure to check the handles against one another to ensure that their overall length is close to uniform.

THE CENTRAL CORD:

This is your 10'-12' section of 7-8mm cord. Tie a double fisherman's knot at each end so that the Klemheist knots cannot accidentally be slid off, and mark the midpoint using your sharpie.

THE PRUSIKS:

Tie your Prusiks as described in ESSENTIAL KNOTS.

Secure them to your central cord using the Klemheist knot, also described in ESSENTIAL KNOTS, each tied so that the wrap moves towards the middle and the final loop points toward the end. Clip your carabiners or utility clips through the loops, and also through the loop of your handle. You have now completed your very own suspension device.

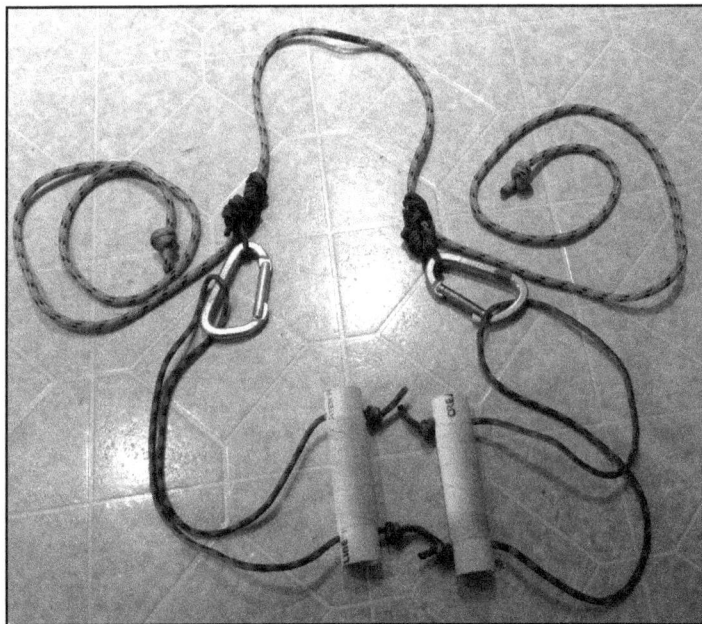

A complete workout program designed to be used with this device follows in PART TWO: YOU AND YOUR SUSPENSION DEVICE: A LOVE / HATE STORY.

PART TWO

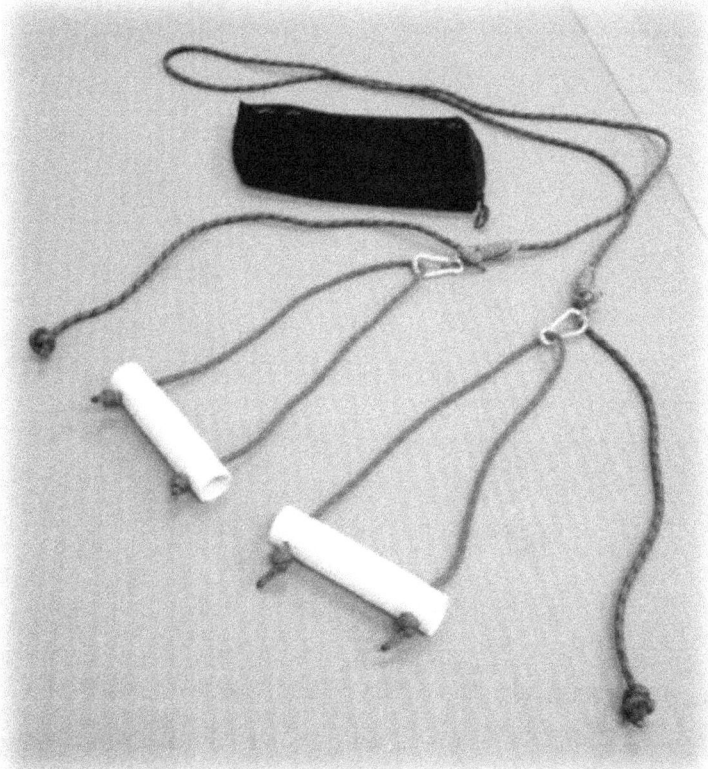

YOU AND YOUR
SUSPENSION DEVICE:
A LOVE / HATE STORY

CONTENTS

TRAINING PHILOSOPHY & APPROACH

The workout contained in this manual is based on the "5 Pillar" model of strength training. Essentially it holds that, on the whole, the human body is designed to enact 5 fundamental movement patters—Vertical Pulling and Pushing, Horizontal Pushing and Pulling, Hingeing, Squatting, and Rotating—and that by exercising a given movement pattern we exercise all of the muscles that work to produce that movement pattern, and in so doing we not only strengthen the body as a whole but also improve motor function and mobility (our ability to get into and out of all natural ranges of motion).

The training protocol I outline in this manual is a Timed Static Contraction (TSC) protocol. Rather than moving through a movement pattern, in the TSC protocol a given movement (a Vertical Pull, for example) is held at full exertion in the midrange of the movement, for time. While this may seem counter-productive to the proposed benefit outlined above (the improvement of motor function and mobility throughout a range of motion), this protocol has in fact been shown to produce full range-of-motion strength, and carries the added benefit of being the simplest protocol to follow (meaning that there is less to keep track of while you're working, thus allowing you to focus on form and engagement). And, once acclimated to the exercises and the workout, the TSC protocol can very easily be substituted out for a more traditional, rep-based workout.

Extensive research done by Dr. Doug McGuff and John Little (outlined in their book BODY BY SCIENCE) suggests that a single set of an exercise performed to the point of temporary muscular failure with a load sufficient to produce muscular failure in not less than 60 but not more than 120 seconds provides the greatest training benefit—a training benefit which is not improved upon by performing multiple failure sets and which is not matched by multiple sub-maximal effort sets (training benefit here being defined as strength gains, stored body fat mobilization, and hormonal changes). **It is therefore our approach in this workout to 1) hold tension (by pulling or pushing against the device) 2) in the midrange of motion for each of the essential pillars of movement 3) for 90 seconds 4) at a level of exertion sufficient to produce temporary muscular failure, (failure here being recognized as the point at which the muscles are unable to produce significant force, manifested either as slacking the tension on the device or involuntarily lowering oneself to the ground, depending on the nature of the movement pillar being exercised).** This protocol will be more throughly explained in the section titled THE WORKOUT.

It should be mentioned also that of all possible training approaches, this is among the safest, if not the safest: handling no external weight and holding with no momentum, it is almost impossible to force a tissue (muscle, tendon, or ligament) to bear more force than it is capable of handling. A tissue that cannot withstand the force it is being asked to produce simply fails to produce that force: you will not find yourself giving out under a heavy bar you can no longer hold, for example. The boon that this offers to an athlete of any age or physical condition cannot be overstated.

THE SUSPENSION DEVICE

The suspension device you made can be employed to work each of the 5 pillars of movement to their absolute limit, and with a little imagination can be employed in dozens of ways for hundreds of exercises. The Klemheist knot which attaches the handles to the central cord is a friction knot which, when unweighted and slightly loosened, will slide freely up and down the length of the central cord but which, when weighted, will tighten around the central cord and stay in place, making the device highly adjustable for a variety of exercises.

The Klemheist Knot

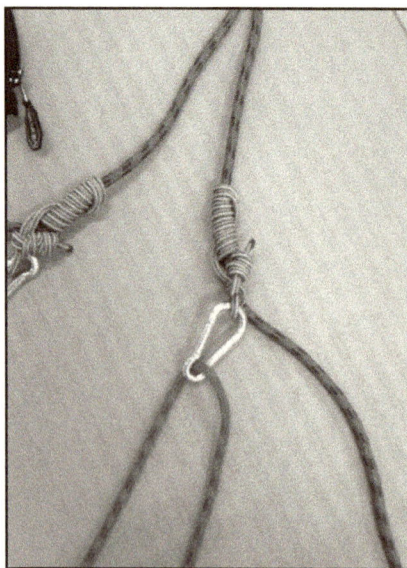

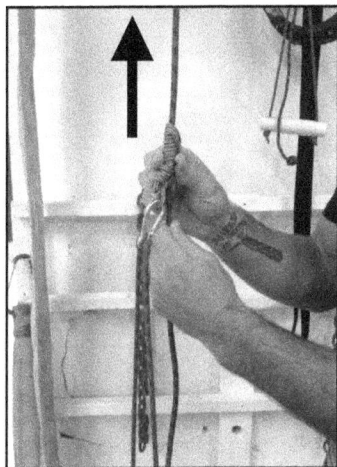

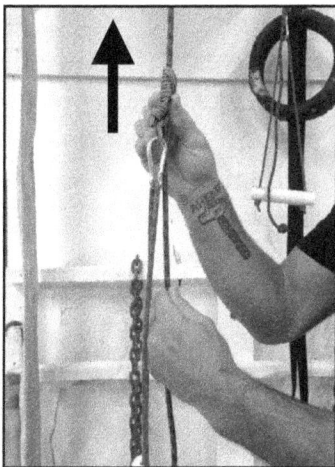

The knot slides easily when slightly loosened and unweighted...

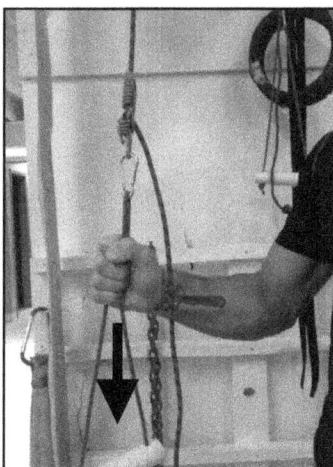

But stays put once it's placed under load.

For some of the exercises outlined in the workout it will be necessary to secure the central cord to a fixed anchor point. A low tree branch, the high bar on a swing set, etc. work well: simply toss one handle over, equalize the ends, and you're ready to go. Without one of these, an average door works in a pinch.

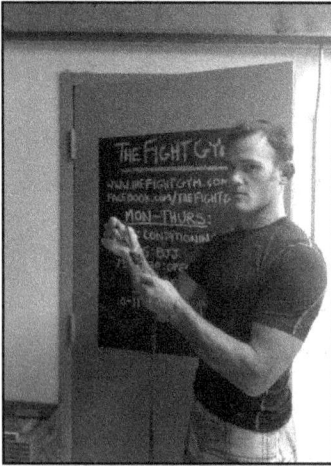

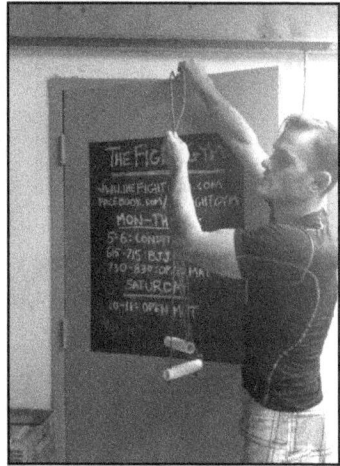

Tie a simple overhand (square) knot at the main cord's midpoint, and pass the knot over the top of the door.

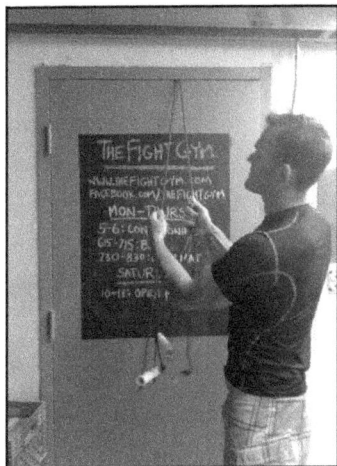

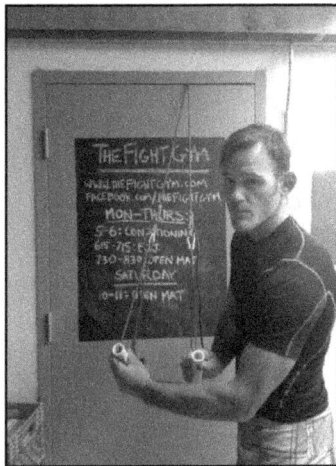

Push the door closed until it latches, and equalize your handles. A latched door should hold your weight with no problem, but it's never a bad idea to set your knot up so that it's pulling against the way the door opens (the opposite of what I've shown here).

THE FIVE PILLARS

As I said in Part 1, the Five Pillars of human movement are: Vertical Pulling and Pushing, Horizontal Pulling and Pushing, Hingeing (Hip-dominant level change), Squatting (Hip- and Knee-dominant level change), and Rotation (or Anti-rotation) of the trunk or spine. Below these movements are illustrated.

Pillar 1: Vertical Push / Pull

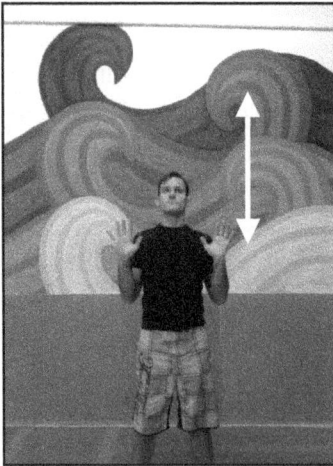

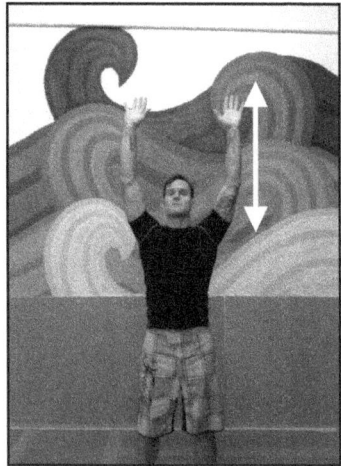

Pillar 2: Horizontal Push / Pull

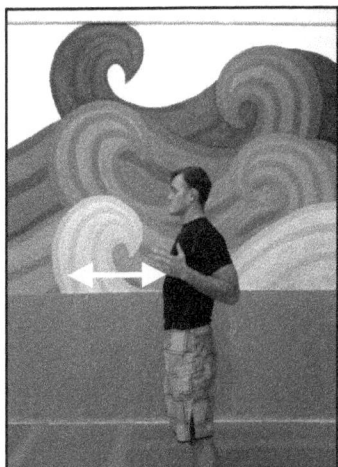

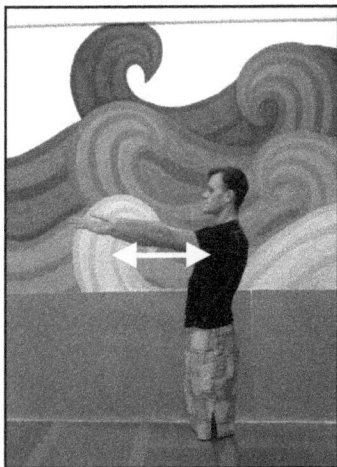

Pillar 3: Squatting. Notice that the knees and shoulders come forward of the center line (the vertical line over the heels) and the hips go back.

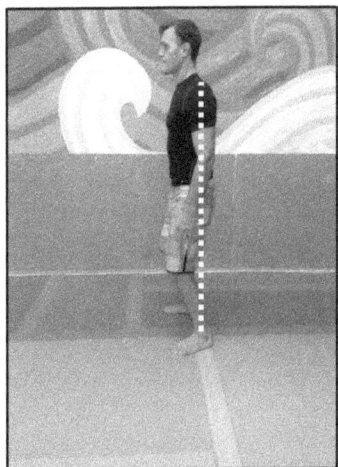

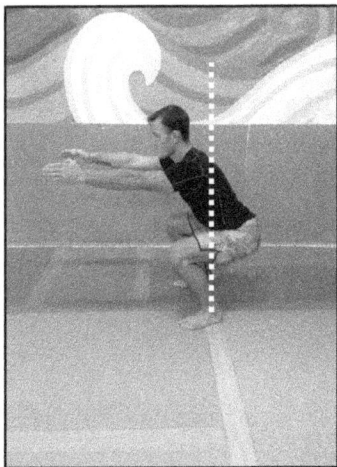

Pillar 4: Hingeing. Note that the shoulders come forward and the hips go back, but the knees stay directly over the ankles.

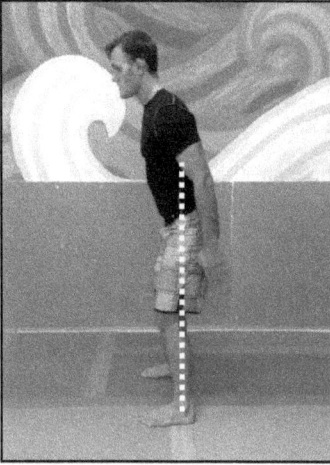

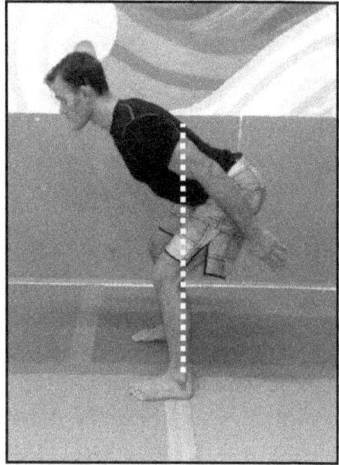

Pillar 5: Rotation / Anti-rotation is most importantly defined by our ability to hold resistance against an offset force attempting to spin our hips and shoulders out of alignment with each other (imagine someone pushing one of your shoulders from the front, such that you would be forced to engage your core to keep your shoulders from turning).

THE WORKOUT

Note: this workout requires that you have a clock visible during each exercise, or that you use an interval timer, interval timer app, or stopwatch.

The workout contained in the following pages should be performed in the following manner. 1) Using the suspension device as shown, place yourself in the midrange for each of the 5 Pillars of movement. 2) Start the clock or timer and begin putting tension into the position, pulling or pushing against the device. There should be no movement, only an increase in tension. Build up the tension slowly and steadily over the course of 30 seconds so that, at the 30 second mark, you are pulling or pushing with near-maximum effort. This first 30-second phase is also the time to "orient" yourself in the position: become aware of the muscles being targeted, check your form, and focus on keeping your breathing steady and controlled (see below). 3) For the next 30 seconds, continue pushing or pulling at this near-maximum level or exertion. Expect that your heart rate will increase and your muscles will burn; this is normal. (Stop immediately if you feel any sharp or sudden pain the the muscles or joints, feel that your heart rate is unusually high, or if you have difficulty breathing.) Attempt to keep constant tension at this level of exertion for the duration of the interval. 4) At the 60-second mark, increase your level of exertion until you are pulling or pushing "as hard as you dare." This phase will be quite uncomfortable (with burning muscles and elevated heart and respiration rate) and you will be tempted to slack and rest, but it is essential that you don't: this final, stressful phase is what signals my body that it must grow stronger. As we are at our most fatigued at this point, it is essential that we remain aware of form, and continue to monitor ourselves. After 30 seconds of this effort (after a total of 90 seconds in the position), gradually ease off over the course of 3-5 seconds. Your session with that pillar is now complete.

A complete workout would consist of one 90-second session of this protocol with each Pillar. Done properly the workout should take no more than 20 minutes (including rest), and will consist of no more than 10.5 minutes of work (1.5 min / exercise). Your personal recovery needs may vary, but for new trainees I recommend performing the workout once every 5-7 days.

And before we begin, a word about the breath: breath should be inhaled through the nose, and may be exhaled through either the nose or the mouth. Breath should be drawn into the diaphragm (belly breathing), but should be done without releasing core tension. For this purpose it is best to take small "sips" of air, letting the tensed abdomen expand slightly, and then once again contracting the abdominal muscles to exhale. This will take some practice, but the benefit of the of the TSC protocol is that, without worrying about counting or moving, we can give the breath our attention. It is essential that you not gasp, gulp, grunt, or hold the breath, as this is at best detrimental to overall health (it causes a cascade of stress responses) and at worst dangerous (it causes a pronounced spike in blood pressure). Breath should be smooth and controlled throughout the interval.

Pillar 1A: The Vertical Pull

Note: The simplest exercise for this pillar is the pull up or chin up. Holding a static chin up for 90 seconds is quite a feat of strength, and I am assuming that we're going to have to work into it. What I've included here are some modifications in which the legs can be used for an assist.

VARIATION 1

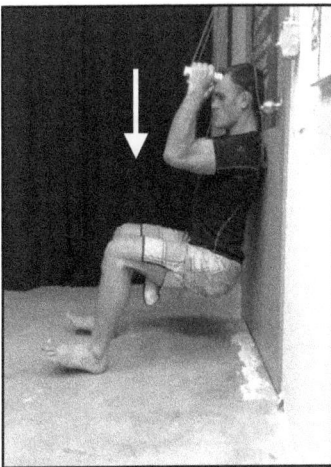

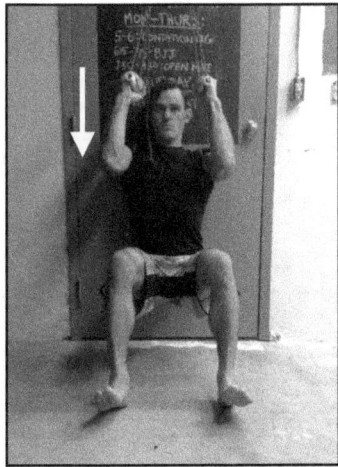

Securing the suspension device in the door, adjust the handles so that you can hang with bent legs and arms bent at 90 degrees. Using your legs as much or as little as needed, attempt to pull yourself up the door. Ideally you should find yourself unable to keep your arms bent, and find yourself slowly sitting down on the floor, at around the 90 second mark. If you find that you can reach 90 seconds with no problem, use your legs less (potentially to the point of picking your feet up off the floor). Notice I am keeping my spine almost completely vertical, so that both my shoulders and my hips are inline (or almost inline) with the door, and that I am flexing my feet upward to keep me from pushing too much with my legs.

VARIATION 2

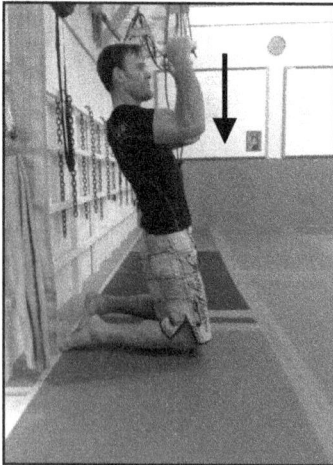

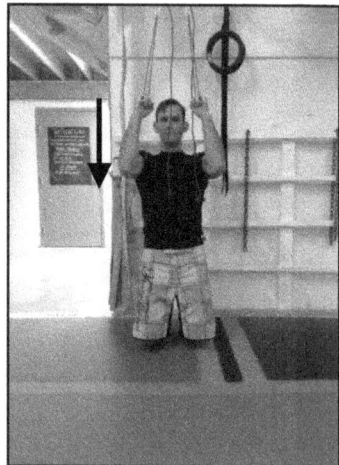

Securing the suspension device over a branch, pull up bar, swing set, etc., I adjust the handles so that, when I kneel directly under the anchor point, I can reach the handles with my arms bent at 90 degrees (upper arms parallel to the ground). I lift my knees off the ground, giving myself minor assistance by pushing off the tops of my feet. Note that even if you are unable to keep your knees off the ground for the duration of the 90 seconds, you should continue to pull as hard as you can until time runs out.

VARIATION 3

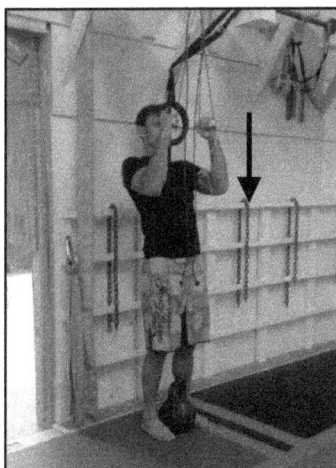

If you have a high anchor and something under which you can secure your feet, you can perform the variation illustrated in the image above. Note that in the imagine I am pinching a kettlebell between my feet. The kettlebell keeps me from being able to pick my feet up off the ground, thus forcing me to stay in the midrange, even though I'm pulling as hard as I can.

Pillar 1B: The Vertical Push

Adjust the suspension device so that when you are standing on the cord you are able to hold the handles with your arms at 90 degrees, upper arms parallel to the ground. It is of paramount importance here that we stabilize the base and lower back: while under tension, isometrically contract the legs, butt, and lower back. Notice that the direction of my push is up and slightly forward, that my chest is open and my spine is slightly arched. Note that, for the sake of comfort, it is preferable to either wear shoes while performing this exercise, or place a towel between the cord and your feet.

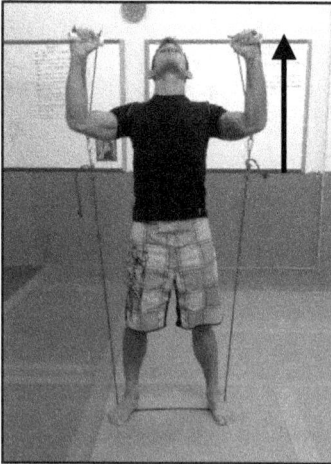

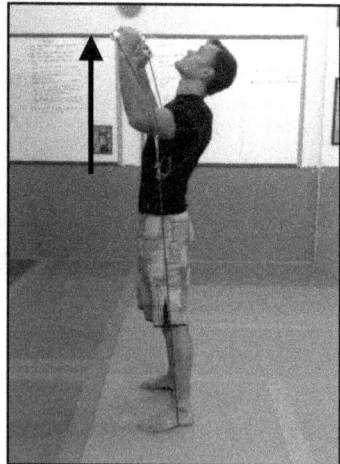

Pillar 2A: The Horizontal Pull

The horizontal pull is your basic row. In the following pages I show two variations for performing this exercise with your suspension device.

VARIATION 1

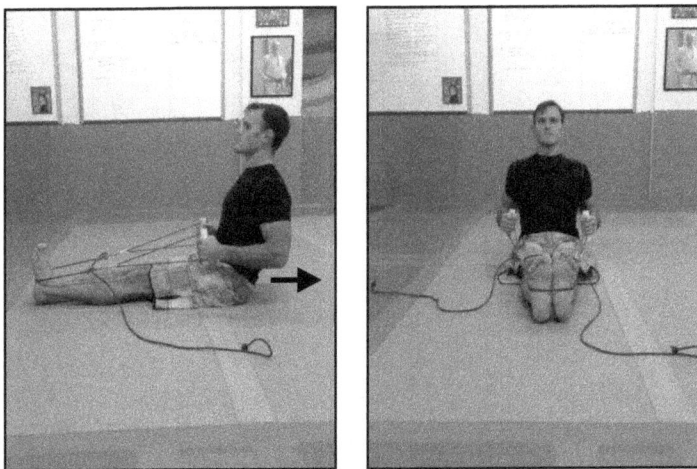

Sit on the floor with your legs and back straight. Pass the central cord around your feet and adjust the length so that you can hold the handles with your arms bent at 90 degrees, upper arms vertical and elbows against the sides. As with the Vertical Push, it is preferable to wear shoes or place a towel between the cord and your feet. For the TSC protocol this option is preferable in some ways to Variation 2, which lends itself well to repetitions of bodyweight rows.

VARIATION 2

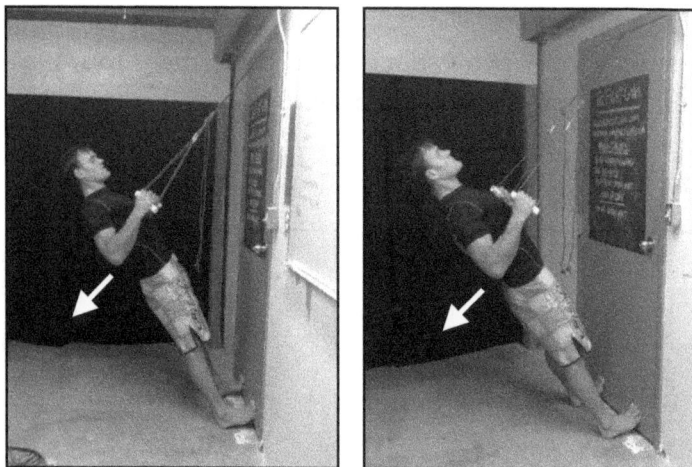

Securing the suspension device in a door, adjust the handles so that, when positioned in the bodyweight row posture, you are handling an appropriate amount of your bodyweight (meaning that you are not at such a low angle that you cannot hold for 90 seconds, or at such a high angle that 90 seconds fails to produce sufficient fatigue. Finding the appropriate angle may take some experimentation). Pull the shoulders down and together behind you, and pull your elbows back and together ("spread" your hands) Once you have pulled yourself into full contraction (the top position), continue to pull as hard as you can, as though to elevate yourself past the handles.

Pillar 2B: The Horizontal Push

The standard exercise for the horizontal push is your basic push up. However, for a TSC protocol, I like to use the suspension device as an impediment, so that try as I might I am unable to push myself up. If this method proves too difficult, I have included a second variation.

VARIATION 1

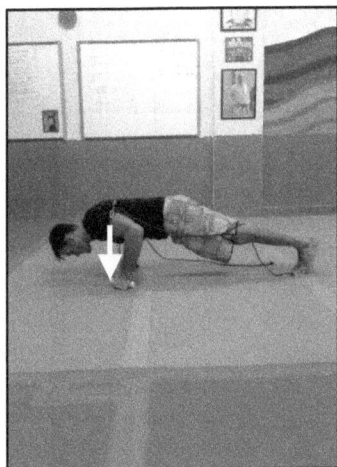

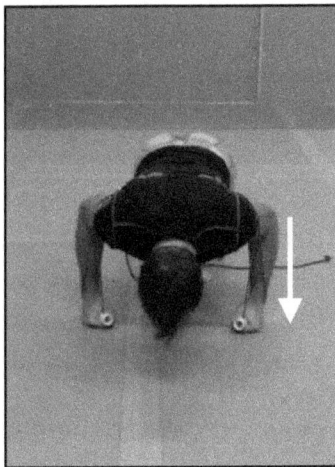

Pass the suspension device behind your upper back and adjust it so that, when holding the handles, your arms cannot extend past 90 degrees and your elbows are at your sides. Place yourself into the push up position and attempt to push up through the cord. Note that, when performing this variation, I tuck my tailbone and round my back into a static hollow body, an addition I will discuss more in the section on Pillar 5.

VARIATION 2

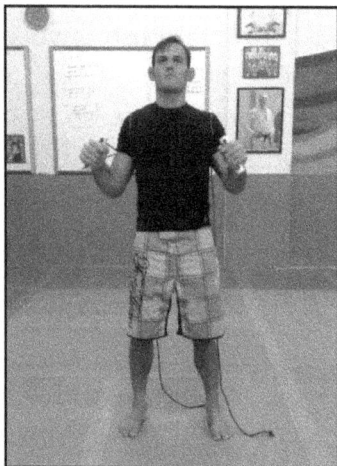

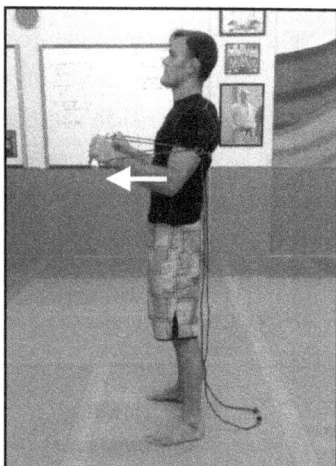

Rigging the suspension device in the same fashion that you would for variation one, remain seated, standing, kneeling, or whatever is comfortable while you push the handles away from you as hard as you can. Note that, for comfort, you may want to wear a heavier sweatshirt or put a towel between the cord and your back.

Pillar 3: Squatting

Note that, for this exercise, you will need to tinker with your device to find the right length. As illustrated in the picture on the following page, the final position should put my torso at 90 degrees to my upper legs and my upper legs at 90 degrees to my lower legs.

1. Wrap the central cord around your waist, as you would a bathrobe belt. 2. Cross the cord in front of you. 3. Squat and place the handles on the ground, and place your feet on the handle cord so that the handle itself is running along the outside edge of your foot. Position yourself so that your knees are bent and moved out over the toes. Back should be arched, chest should be out, shoulder blades should be pulled back and together, head should be up. Legs must be parallel. Essentially you attempt to stand up through the cord. The effort should be felt primarily in the front thighs, but the glutes, hamstrings, and calves are also involved. Note that you may want to place a towel between your waist and the cord.

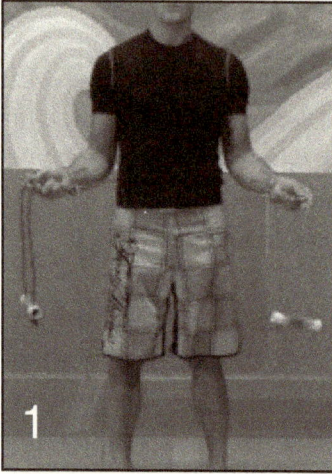
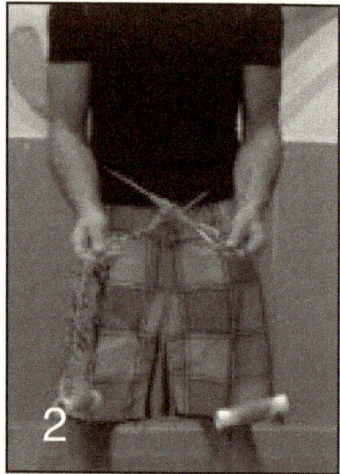
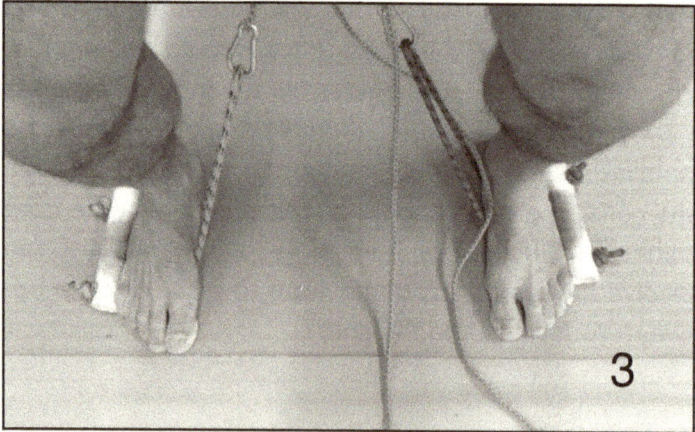

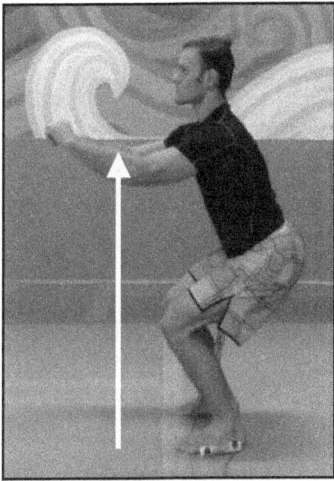

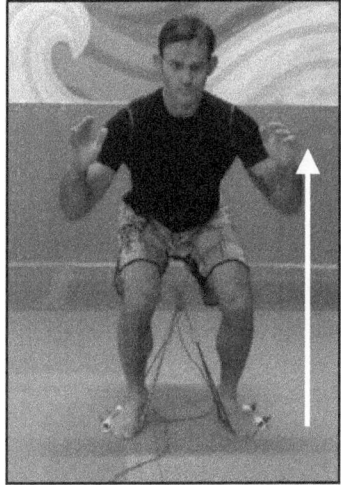

In the squat, the legs drive the hips and shoulders straight up.

Pillar 4: Hingeing

Adjust the device so that, when standing on the central cord, the handles reach up to knee height. Bend at the waist, dropping the hips back and letting the shoulders come forward, bending slightly at the knees so that the shins remain vertical. Back should be arched, chest should be out, shoulder blades should be pulled back and together, head should be in line with the rest of the spine. Feet should be hip width and legs must be parallel. Again you attempt to stand up through the cord, although this time the primary action is of rising from a bow. The effort should be felt primarily in the glutes and hamstrings, but the front thighs are also involved. Note that, as with the vertical push, you may want to wear shoes or place a towel between your feet and the cord.

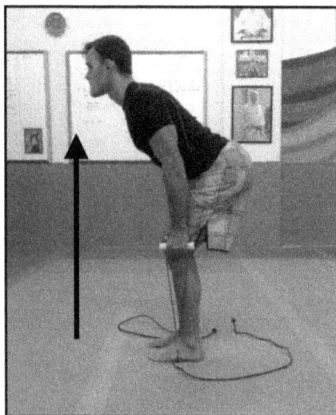

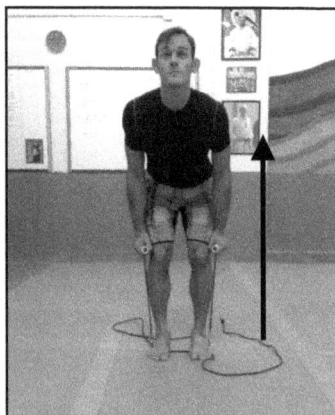

In the hinge the gluteals drive the hips forward. Shoulders go back. Body "unfolds" like a jackknife.

46

Pillar 5: Rotation / Anti-rotation (a.k.a. Core Stability)

The purpose of the core is to stabilize the spine. The arch in the back on the hinge and the squat work the muscles of the back that provide stability there. The "hollow-body plank" is designed to work the series of muscles that join the pelvis to the ribcage on the front side.

Get down into an elbow plank (push up position, but with your arms bent so that you are resting on your forearms and elbows). Round your back and isometrically contract your abs, like you're doing a crunch. You can think about attempting to pull your elbows towards your toes and your toes towards your elbows. I like to also work this "hollow body" position into my horizontal push (the push up position).

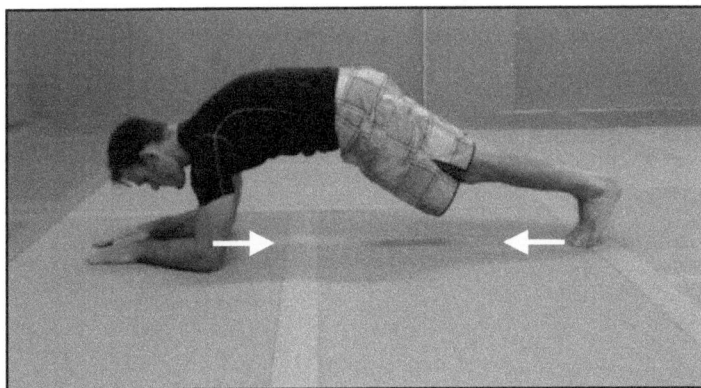

So to recap: the workout would include 90 seconds of effort at the midrange point for each of the 5 Pillars of Human Movement for a total of 10.5 minutes of work, performed once every 5-7 days. The 5 pillars and their corresponding exercises are listed below in the order in which I usually perform them in my own workouts.

Vertical Pull (Pull Up)
Vertical Push (Overhead Press)
Squat (Squat)
Horizontal Pull (Row)
Horizontal Press (Push Up)
Hinge (Dead Lift)
Anti-rotation (Hollow-body Plank)

You can let me know how you like the program and what kind of results you see on Facebook, either through my author page (@ScottBurrAuthor) or the Superhero Simplified page (@SuperheroSimplified).

Thanks for reading. I wish you good luck and good training.

Stay super,

Scott Burr

ABOUT THE AUTHOR

Scott Burr is a graduate of the creative writing program at The Colorado College, where he was co-chair of the Climber's Association of Colorado College (CACC) and head route-setter at the Ritt Kellogg Climbing Gym.

A long-time martial artist, Scott holds black belt rank in Gracie Jiu-Jitsu, Kodokan Judo, and the Korean art of Kuk Sul Do. He has also trained extensively in Muay Thai, Boxing, and Submission Grappling, and has trained with and learned from some of the top names in combat sports, including many members of the Gracie Family.

Scott is a certified pro fitness trainer under legendary strength & conditioning coach Steve Maxwell. He holds additional MaxwellSC certifications in Kettlebell (Level 1 and 2) and Bodyweight (Level 1 and 2) training. He has traveled internationally with Steve, assisting at seminars on everything from kettlebell training to joint mobility to breathwork.

Scott was the head instructor and head strength & conditioning coach at The Fight Gym, a Gracie Jiu-Jitsu school and fitness facility located outside Cleveland, Ohio, for over a decade.

Scott is the author of the novels *Bummed Out City* and *We Will Rid the World of You*, and the essay collection

Superhero Simplified: Collected, Selected, Revised and Expanded. He is also the author of the training manual *Get a Grip: A Practical Primer on Grip Strength and Endurance Training… and More.* His short stories and novel excerpts have appeared *Metonym, Mildred, The Decades Review*, and elsewhere. His nonfiction has been published in Climbing and Urban Climber magazines.

Scott is the 2002 winner of the Ebey Prize for novella-length fiction and was a finalist for the 2004 Reville Prize in short fiction. He is also the 2006 winner of the Geauga Park District Foundation Nature Writing Contest, and was a finalist for the Gordon Square Review's inaugural contest for Northeast Ohio writers (2017). His novel *Bummed Out City* was one of Library Journal's most-read books for 2015.

Scott is currently head of design for Hold Fast Grip Tech, where he is refining and improving the training gadgets he dreamed up and developed over his years as the head strength & conditioning coach at The Fight Gym. Visit HoldFastGripTech.com to learn more.

If you are interested in training with Scott, or would like to inquire about hosting a seminar with Scott at your facility, contact information may be found at www.EnclaveJiuJitsu.com.